Senior Strength: Enhance Stability, Prevent Falls, and Boost Posture with Easy At-Home Workouts

<u>*Description*</u>

The indispensable manual "Senior Strength: Improve Posture, Prevent Falls, and Enhance Stability with Simple At-Home Exercises" is designed to assist you in attaining and sustaining a dynamic and active way of life during your golden years.

 It is a normal process to undergo bodily changes with age, such as diminished bone density, equilibrium problems, and a reduction in muscle mass; these changes can elevate the risk of falls and negatively impact our quality of life. This eBook serves as an all-encompassing resource for seniors seeking safe and effective at-home workouts that specifically target these concerns. You will discover a multitude of expert advice, clear and concise workout routines, and helpful hints on nutrition and lifestyle modifications within these pages. Gain insights into improving your posture, preventing accidents, and enhancing your stability with the assistance of straightforward exercises tailored to suit individuals of different fitness levels. Significant progress can be made from the convenience of one's own residence, without the need for costly gym memberships or specialized apparatus. By adhering to the recommendations outlined in "Senior Strength," one will not only gain increased self-assurance in their physical maneuvers but also encounter heightened vitality and autonomy. Age should not be an impediment to experiencing life to the utmost. Using this empowering eBook, initiate the process of attaining a state of improved health, strength, and equilibrium. Your future self will be extremely appreciative.

Table of Contents

Introduction

1. Introduce the Importance of Balance for Seniors.

The Importance of Balance for Seniors

When people become older, it is more important than ever before for their general health and quality of life that they have a healthy balance in their lives. When it comes to one's physical health, balance is a crucial component that is often disregarded until it shows signs of deterioration. When it comes to seniors, keeping their balance is important more than simply preventing falls; it's also about maintaining their independence, mobility, mental well-being, and general health. We will dig into the different elements of this problem and give insights into how seniors may develop and maintain their balance for a happier and more satisfying life as part of our complete investigation of the relevance of balance for elders.

The Aging Process and Balance

The process of ageing is a natural and unavoidable component of life, and as we get older, our physiques go through a lot of changes. A good number of these shifts have an influence on our capacity to efficiently maintain equilibrium. The following is a list of some of the most important age-related issues that might affect balance:

Strength and Mass of the Muscles: Sarcopenia is the medical period for the gradual loss of both muscular strength and mass that occurs naturally with advancing age. The inability to regulate their motions and keep their balance might be impacted by the natural decline in muscular strength that comes with ageing.

Flexibility in the Joints: As people become older, they often experience a stiffening of the joints. When joint flexibility is reduced, it may be challenging to maintain balance, particularly when it comes to making fast changes to avoid falling over.

Sensory Perception: alterations in eyesight and the vestibular system, which are both affected by ageing, play a role in maintaining our feeling of balance. Ageing may lead to a reduction in sensory perception, including these alterations. Because of these changes, there is a potential increase in the risk of falling.

Reaction Time: As we become older, it takes us longer to respond appropriately to unanticipated challenges, such as a shift in our equilibrium or an unexpected obstruction. Seniors, who often have longer response times, may be more prone to falling as a result.

Chronic Health Issues Chronic health issues, such as diabetes, cardiovascular illness, and arthritis, may influence a person's balance and increase the risk of falling. Seniors are more prone to these diseases than younger people.

Medicine: a significant number of elderly people use medicine that, among other side effects, may produce dizziness, sleepiness, or variations in blood pressure, all of which can contribute to issues with balance.

The Consequences of Poor Balance in Seniors

Why is it so crucial for seniors to maintain their equilibrium, and what are the repercussions of failing to do so? Let's take a look at some of the possible consequences that might result from an older adult's life having an imbalance:

Increased danger of Falls: The heightened danger of falling is the most pressing worry at this time. Falls are a prominent cause of injury-related hospitalization and even mortality among people in this age range, making them a significant problem for public health in the elderly population. Fractures, brain injuries, and other forms of severe trauma are common outcomes for senior citizens who suffer from falls.

Loss of Independence: Loss of independence may result from poor balance, which can lead to falling. The fear of elderly people falling might cause them to restrict their activities and level of involvement in everyday life, which can result in a worse quality of life.

Reduced movement: The ability to keep one's balance is very necessary for movement. When your equilibrium is off, it may be difficult for you to walk, climb stairs, and carry out other tasks that are part of your daily routine.

Confidence and Mental Health: Issues with one's balance might make one less confident in one's own physical ability, which can have a negative impact on one's mental health. This decline in self-confidence may be a factor in social isolation, anxiety, and depression.

Injury: Seniors who have poor balance are more prone to experience injuries beyond falls, as their general capacity to defend themselves from mishaps weakens. These injuries may include broken bones and head trauma.

Cognitive Decline: There is some evidence from research that suggests that activities that stress one's balance, such as balance training, might have a beneficial effect on cognitive performance. This is of utmost significance since cognitive decline is a major reason for anxiety among those in their older years.

Preventing Falls and Maintaining Balance

It is crucial to take preventative action with regard to this problem, given the fundamental relevance of balance for elderly citizens. The following is a list of numerous tactics and approaches that may assist older citizens in avoiding falling and keeping their balance:

Regular Exercise: Participating in regular physical exercise is one of the most effective methods to maintain and develop your balance, and it is also one of the most enjoyable ones. Tai chi, yoga, and Pilates are three examples of exercises that may be quite useful. These kinds of workouts aim to improve strength, flexibility, and balance.

Strength Training: Workouts that focus on building and maintaining muscular strength are essential for keeping a healthy balance. Seniors may improve their balance and stability by participating in strength training activities that focus on their primary muscle groups.

Training for Flexibility: Stretching exercises may enhance joint flexibility, which enables seniors to make essential changes more easily and maintain balance more successfully.

Balance Training: Training the Body to keep Its Balance The capacity to keep one's balance may be considerably improved by including particular balancing exercises as part of one's everyday regimen. These exercises could take standing on one leg, trying to maintain balance on an unsteady surface, or walking heel-to-toe in a circle.

Proper Footwear: Footwear that is Appropriate For Maintaining Balance Keeping your balance requires you to wear shoes that are both supportive and fit properly. Slips and falls are easier to avoid while wearing shoes with non-slip soles.

Home Safety Measures: Seniors may lessen the danger of falling in their own homes by clearing away clutter, fastening carpets, adding grab bars in restrooms, and making sure there is enough lighting.

Medication Management: Seniors should speak with their healthcare professionals about their medicines in order to have an understanding of any possible adverse effects that might influence their sense of balance. It's possible that your drug schedule may need some tweaking.

Regular Vision and Hearing Checks: Examining the Eyes and Ears on a Regular Basis Carrying out regular eye and ear tests may assist seniors in maintaining their sensory perception and addressing any abnormalities that may impact their balance.

Hydration and Nutrition: It is possible to make a contribution to one's general health and well-being by keeping a balanced diet and drinking an adequate amount of water. This will indirectly assist balance.

Consult with Healthcare Professionals: Physical therapists and occupational therapists are trained to diagnose balance problems and create individualized workout plans to treat them. If it is required, they are also able to provide instruction on the use of assistive technologies.

Promoting a Holistic Approach to Senior Balance

A holistic approach to maintaining elders' balance and preventing falls requires taking into consideration not just the physical components of maintaining balance but also its psychological, social, and mental dimensions as well. Consider the following important aspects of the situation:

Emotional Well-Being: The worry that one would hurt oneself by falling can have a considerable negative effect on a senior's mental health. It's possible that fostering a constructive mindset and assisting elders in overcoming their anxieties might be just as vital as encouraging physical activity.

Social Engagement: Seniors who continue to have active social lives are more likely to be physically active and emotionally resilient than their peers who do not. It is possible to have a beneficial effect on the well-being of older citizens by encouraging them to participate in social activities.

Engaging the Brain: Cognitive performance may be improved by the practice of balance exercises that provide a challenge to the brain. The practice of dance may improve cognitive health, the acquisition of new abilities, and the playing of games that challenge the mind.

Individualized Method: The requirements and difficulties of ageing are different for each and every senior. It is very necessary for success to adapt balancing programs to the specific capabilities and concerns of each person.

Regular Evaluation: It is vital to conduct regular evaluations of one's balance and fall risk. Changes may be recognized by medical professionals, who can then respond appropriately.

The Role of Healthcare Providers

It is the responsibility of healthcare professionals to assist elderly patients in maintaining their balance and avoiding falls. The following is how they may make a contribution:

Education: Healthcare providers may educate older patients about the significance of maintaining their balance as well as the preventative measures they can take to reduce their risk of falling.

Assessment: Regular evaluations of one's balance and potential for falling may assist in the early detection of problems and the formulation of treatment strategies.

Physical therapy: Physical therapists may help elders improve their balance and build exercise regimens that are specifically catered to the requirements of older adults.

Medication Review: assess medicines. Healthcare professionals may assess patients' medicines to see if any of them may impact their balance and then make any necessary changes.

Referral to experts: In situations when balance problems are connected to certain medical disorders, healthcare practitioners may send senior patients to experts for further assessment and treatment. Referrals to specialists can be made for both diagnostic and therapeutic purposes.

Technological Advancements for Senior Balance

Because of advances in technology, older people now have access to new tools and services that may assist them in keeping their equilibrium. The following are some examples:

Wearable Devices: Balance and fall detection functions are often included in fitness trackers and smartwatches that are designed to be worn. These gadgets are capable of providing data in real-time and even sending notifications if they detect a fall.

Virtual Reality (VR) and Exergaming: Both virtual reality systems and exergaming platforms provide users with strategies to enhance their balance that are both interactive and interesting. These technologies may make balancing workouts more pleasurable, which will promote consistency and continued participation.

Telehealth: As telehealth services grow easier to obtain, they make it possible for older citizens to consult with medical professionals and physical therapists via remote means. Those individuals who may have problems getting to medical institutions may find this to be an especially helpful resource.

Conclusion

A senior's physical, emotional, social, and mental well-being are all included in the concept of balance, which is an essential component of senior health. The ability to keep one's balance is critical for seniors to have in order to reduce the risk of falling, retain their independence, continue to be mobile, increase their confidence, and ensure their general health and vitality. It is a comprehensive strategy that needs a mix of different things, such as physical activity, changes to one's lifestyle, the installation of safety measures in one's house, and assistance from medical specialists. Taking care of one's balance and preventing falls as one gets older should not be seen as an afterthought but rather as an essential component of ageing gracefully and experiencing a good quality of life. It is important for elders, their families, and the healthcare experts who care for them to collaborate in order to emphasize finding a healthy balance in their lives. This will ensure that seniors continue to enjoy life to the fullest. Seniors may traverse the process of ageing with elegance and self-assurance if they take preventative measures to develop and maintain their sense of equilibrium.

Chapter 1: Understanding Balance

1. Discuss the Physical and Mental Aspects of Balance.

The Physical and Mental Aspects of Balance

The idea of balance may be broken down into its component parts, which include both the physical and the mental aspects. It has a significant effect on our day-to-day lives, having a bearing not only on our bodily steadiness but also on our coordination and mobility, as well as our mental well-being and our capacity for thought. During this investigation of the physical and mental components of balance, we will dig into the interaction between these two dimensions and the relevance they have for general health and quality of life. Specifically, we will focus on how the mind and body affect each other.

Physical Aspects of Balance

The capacity of the body to keep its equilibrium, regulate its movements, and avoid falling is the primary meaning of the term "physical balance." It involves the intricate cooperation of many of the body's internal systems. The following is a list of some of the most important physical characteristics of balance:

Vestibular System: Vestibular System The vestibular system, which is responsible for sensing changes in head position and movement, is housed in the inner ear. It assists us in keeping our sense of balance, which is especially beneficial during activities such as walking and jogging.

Muscle Power and Coordination: The power of our muscles and their capacity to function together in harmony is very necessary for maintaining our physical equilibrium. Not only do muscles provide the essential power for movement, but they also assist in the stabilization of our joints and the maintenance of our posture.

Proprioception: The capacity of our body to perceive the position and movement of our individual body parts is referred to as proprioception. It is dependent on the particular receptors that are found in the joints, tendons, and muscles. Even when our eyes are closed, we are able to keep our equilibrium because of a sense called proprioception, which enables us to make changes in our subconscious.

Flexibility in the Joints: The degree to which our joints are pliable determines the range of motion we are capable of, which in turn affects our overall balance. Joints that are stiff may restrict mobility and make the body less stable.

Time to React: Being able to react quickly to shifts in balance is essential for reducing the risk of falling. This needs the neurological system, the muscles, and the sensory organs to work in concert with one another.

Visual Perception: Vision is an important component of balance because it enables us to assess our surroundings and make the required modifications in order to navigate around obstacles and preserve our sense of equilibrium.

Somatosensory System: The somatosensory system is the part of the body that processes information about touch and pressure. It is extremely important for us to keep this muscle strong when our vision is poor since it helps us keep our balance.

A person's physical equilibrium is not a fixed quality; rather, it is dynamic and may change over time. It makes it possible for humans to adapt to a wide variety of motions and activities, ranging from simple ones like walking and climbing stairs to more complicated ones. When our bodily equilibrium is off, we increase our risk of falling, which may lead to injuries and make it more difficult for us to carry out the tasks of daily living.

Mental Aspects of Balance

The mental side of balance is related to our emotional, psychological, and cognitive well-being, in contrast to the physical aspect of balance, which refers to the equilibrium of our bodies. A person is said to be in a condition of mental balance when they are in a state of equilibrium in which they are emotionally stable, psychologically well-off, and cognitively harmonious. The following are some essential components of maintaining mental equilibrium:

Emotional control and Stability: Emotional control and stability are both components of mental equilibrium. It encompasses the capacity to control and react to a wide range of emotions, including stress, anxiety, anger, and grief, in a healthy and adaptable way.

Psychological Well-Being: Emotional and mental equilibrium are inextricably related to one another. Psychological well-being is characterized by a number of characteristics, including a positive attitude toward life, the capacity to successfully deal with adversity, and high levels of self-esteem and acceptance of oneself.

Resilience: A person who is psychologically well-balanced has a greater tendency to be more resilient when confronted with hardship. They are able to recover from failures, adjust well to new circumstances, and keep their feeling of inner balance even while facing difficult circumstances.

Cognitive Harmony: The concept of mental equilibrium also includes the concept of cognitive harmony. It requires the capacity for clear thinking, the ability to make judgments, and the ability to retain attention and focus. People who have a healthy mental balance often have a sophisticated and flexible mental capacity.

Relationships and other forms of social interaction: In general, a person who has achieved mental equilibrium is better able to create and sustain good relationships. They are able to speak clearly, exhibit empathetic behaviour, and establish productive social bonds.

Stress Management: Maintaining a state of mental equilibrium is essential to practicing good stress management. Those who have mental equilibrium are better able to deal with the pressures of everyday life without succumbing to crippling anxiety or suffering any of the other adverse consequences that might result from this.

Mental equilibrium is not a fixed condition; rather, it is a dynamic and ever-evolving component of one's overall health and well-being. It is possible for a variety of circumstances, including one's life experiences, level of social support, methods of coping, and individual personality features, to have an effect on it. It is possible for a person to improve their entire quality of life and contribute to a better level of life satisfaction by achieving and maintaining mental equilibrium.

The Interplay between Physical and Mental Balance

The mental and physical components of equilibrium are inextricably linked, and the ways in which they mutually affect one another are manifold:

Physical Well-Being Affects Mental Well-Being: When a person is confronted with physical discomfort, pain, or restrictions as a result of poor balance or other health difficulties, it is possible for this to have a substantial influence on their psychological well-being. This is due to the fact that physical well-being affects mental well-being. For example, those who live with chronic pain may have increased levels of anxiety and despair, as well as a decline in their overall quality of life.

Mental Well-Being Impacts Physical Health: The state of one's mental health may have an effect on one's physical health, and mental equilibrium is a factor in the achievement of favourable health outcomes. People who have lower stages of stress, anxiety, and depression often have greater immune function and lower overall stages of inflammation in their bodies. These elements have the potential to impact one's physical balance by lowering the risk of conditions that have an effect on the musculoskeletal system and general mobility.

Cognitive Function and Balance: Cognitive Function and Physical equilibrium Maintaining cognitive harmony is very necessary for maintaining one's physical equilibrium. It is much easier for a person to receive sensory information and respond fast to keep their bodily balance when they are able to think clearly, make judgments, and retain their attention when they have these abilities.

Emotional Regulation and Response to Falls: The degree to which a person is able to maintain their equilibrium emotionally has a direct bearing on how they react to the experience of falling or to other challenges to their physical equilibrium. Those who are better able to regulate their emotions may recover from their illness more rapidly and approach their rehabilitation with a more optimistic frame of mind.

Adaptability and Resilience: Adaptability, a component of mental balance, is needed for adjusting to changes in physical capacities. Resilience is a component of mental balance. For example, elderly people may have trouble maintaining physical balance as a result of ageing, but their ability to remain resilient and maintain mental equilibrium might help them adapt to these changes more efficiently.

Social support: from Others, The quality of an individual's mental health has an effect on the social interactions and connections that person has. In turn, having social support may have a favourable influence on one's physical equilibrium. Participating in activities that promote both one's physical and mental health, such as group fitness courses, for instance, might be beneficial.

Strategies for Enhancing Both Physical and Mental Balance

Engaging in Regular Physical Activity: Participating in regular exercise, particularly those that focus on improving balance, may help improve both a person's physical and mental equilibrium. Pilates, yoga, and tai chi are examples of exercises that are designed to improve physical stability while also fostering emotional and psychological well-being.

Meditation and Mindfulness: The practices of mindfulness and meditation may assist people in developing the ability to better regulate their emotions and become more resilient. These techniques may have a beneficial influence on one's mental equilibrium and decrease stress, both of which can lead to improvements in one's physical equilibrium.

Adequate Nutrition: Both your physical and mental health may benefit from consuming a diet that is well-balanced. Consuming meals that are high in various nutrients nourishes both the body and the mind, which contributes to an improved sense of well-being.

Strategies for Managing Stress: Learning and practising strategies for managing stress, such as deep breathing, progressive muscle relaxation, and time management, may lessen the harmful influence that stress has on both a person's physical and mental equilibrium.

Social Engagement: Participation in social activities. Keeping social connections and healthy interactions is critical for maintaining mental equilibrium. Participating in group activities or spending time with friends and family members may make a positive contribution to one's emotional well-being and give chances for physical activities that boost one's sense of balance.

Cognitive Training: Engaging in activities that challenge the mind, such as puzzles, memory games, and learning new abilities, may promote cognitive harmony, enhancing both physical and mental balance. This can be accomplished via cognitive training.

Professional Guidance: Consulting with Healthcare Providers, Physical Therapists, and Mental Health Professionals may give personalized direction for treating Physical and Mental Balance difficulties. Consulting with Healthcare Providers, Physical Therapists, and Mental Health Professionals can give personalized direction for treating physical and mental balance difficulties.

Conclusion

The dynamic relationship between one's mental and physical equilibrium is a crucial but intricate component of one's total health and well-being. When one of the dimensions is damaged, it is possible that the other dimension will also be harmed. Both dimensions influence and support one another. As a result, fixing issues with one's physical balance may have a beneficial effect on one's mental equilibrium and vice versa. For the sake of encouraging a holistic approach to health and well-being, it is vital to get an understanding of the delicate link that exists between mental and physical equilibrium. Persons are able to lead lives that are more meaningful and balanced by implementing tactics that promote both their physical and mental equilibrium. This results in an improvement in the person's quality of life as well as their overall happiness.

Chapter 2: Assessing Your Balance

1. Provide Guidance on Self-Assessing.

Self-Assessment: How To Evaluate Your Performance

Are you looking for a way to identify your strengths and skills? Whether you're just starting out in the industry and looking for ways to advance your skills, or you're currently working in the sector and want to know where you can become better, this guide is for you. You may learn more about your abilities, how they relate to your profession, and any aptitudes you might have by doing an honest evaluation of yourself. Let's take a look at self-assessments, how to do one, and the potential advantages they have for individuals like you.

Key Takeaways

- Self-evaluations are useful tools that may be given to students as well as professionals working in the field. These assessments can be used to understand more about oneself.
- When making decisions about your future, such as choosing a major or switching occupations, do an honest evaluation of yourself first.
- There is a large selection of free self-assessments accessible online in a number of formats.

How To Complete a Self-Assessment

Self-assessments may take many forms, and each form has its own unique information to provide. If you are a student who is having trouble deciding what to study, doing a self-assessment may be a really helpful method to offer yourself some direction and find out what you should be focusing on. Self-evaluation may be used by either a job applicant or an employee to identify whether or not they are a suitable match for the workplace.

Student Self-Assessments

Questions on the things that a student enjoys doing, such as writing, working with their hands, or advising others, are often included in interest tests administered to pupils. Other evaluations may help you determine your values, personality, needs, and goals, which will give insights into your interests. You may then utilize these insights to choose a subject of study that aligns with your interests.

Other methods of evaluating oneself Make advantage of your knowledge and research to examine your:

- Competencies, drives, and interests that are important to the business world
- A sense of belonging to certain corporate cultures
- the manner of leadership

- one's capabilities and gifts
- Individual passions, as well as Unique interests, and how they connect to the work world
- Career Self-Assessments

Even those who are already established in their professions or positions might benefit from doing a self-evaluation. Because persons who have work experience have a greater array of abilities, these exams will be somewhat different from those that students utilize. If you aren't happy with the path you're currently on in your professional life, doing a self-evaluation will help you find any abilities you have that can be applicable to a different employment and career path that would be a better match for you. The original recruiting process, as well as hiring or promoting from inside an organization, may also make use of evaluation tools, many of which can forecast how well an employee would do on the job. These are the following:

Assessments of cognitive ability, including linguistic, mathematical, and reading comprehension skills, among others

Tests of job knowledge: measure what an employee already knows in terms of the skills required to do a job.

Tests of background: personal attributes or hobbies that relate to occupational responsibilities are called biodata tests.

Tips for Self-Assessments

Certain characteristics, such as a person's honesty, reliability, and trustworthiness, are evaluated as part of the integrity process.

Timeliness

Learning about yourself as a person is the goal of doing a self-assessment. To that purpose, I have compiled a list of suggestions for optimizing the outcomes of your self-evaluation, which may be seen below.

A sense of timing

Taking some time to do an evaluation of yourself is often a good idea, particularly if you are interested in learning more about who you are. Having said that, there are circumstances in which it makes even more sense to finish one. Before choosing a concentration for your studies at university, it is a smart move to take at least one — and preferably more than one — of the available evaluations. At the same time, it is also a smart move to evaluate your transferable abilities before leaving your current line of work.

Research Your Options

Although many career and aptitude tests are available for free online or via the career centre of your college or university, some institutions do charge a fee for more in-depth testing. Testing is a component of the application process that certain other firms offer. For instance, 88 of the Fortune 100 businesses have employed the Myers-Briggs Personality Test in their hiring processes.

Note

The O*Net Interest Profiler, which is based on The Holland Code, and the career question on Princetonreview.com are both examples of assessment tools that may be tried out. On the website CareerOneStop, maintained by the United States Department of Labor, users may take a number of free tests, including a skill-matcher exam and an interest assessment. You may input your current job title to see a list of occupations that are similar to your present one in the area devoted to career matching. In addition to this, it provides a cross-reference of your greatest talents against a list of vocations that fit them.

Integrity and candor

When completing a self-assessment test, it's natural to want to put your best foot forward and show off your skills. Having said that, it is necessary to be as honest as you possibly can. If you respond to all of the questions in a manner that you "think" they should be answered or in a manner that does not represent how you feel, then the test is invalidated. If you are dishonest with your responses, the evaluation will provide a conclusion that is not relevant to the circumstances of your life.

Think about it.

Spend some time thinking about how the findings of the self-assessment affect you. Think about the first responses that you had to the findings. Has anything in particular taken you aback? What new insights did you get about who you are? In what ways can you put this information to use in the future? The next step is to consider how to put the findings into action, such as by making adjustments, doing further research, or establishing brand-new objectives. It is possible that you may need to rethink your subsequent actions or consult with someone who knows who can offer information on what capabilities or resources you need to proceed.

The Value of Doing Your Own Evaluation

The most important advantage of doing an honest evaluation of oneself is the development of a deeper comprehension of one's own identity. Despite the fact that this may seem to be self-evident, it has the potential to bring about great growth and adjustments in your life. Take, for instance, that you are now in the second year of your undergraduate studies. You are now majoring in biology with the intention of working in the medical field someday. After you've finished with your general education requirements, you're taking a few courses that are linked to your major, but you're having trouble. You don't find the subject to be intriguing, and as a result, you have trouble learning and remembering all of the information. Instead of continuing along a route that isn't right for you, you might think about doing a self-assessment to find out where else your skills and interests could be more applicable.

The Bottom Line

Personal development may be greatly aided by using self-evaluations as a useful tool. The more you discover about your aptitudes, talents, areas of weakness, and abilities, the more you'll be able to lead yourself toward a lifestyle and line of work that are a good fit for you.

Chapter 3: Benefits of Balance Exercises

1. Highlight the Numerous Advantages of Improving balance.

Enhancing one's balance is an essential component of both improving one's physical fitness and one's general well-being. The capacity to keep one's equilibrium when one is moving or standing still is what we refer to as balance, and it is an essential component in many aspects of our day-to-day lives, from the most fundamental actions like walking and standing to the more sophisticated endeavours like playing sports and working out. In this piece, we will discuss the many benefits that come with cultivating better balance, as well as the reasons why doing so is a necessary component of a healthy way of life. We will explain the positive effects that improved balance may have on your body, mind, and emotions, as well as provide you with some useful advice and exercises to help you attain it.

1. Injury Prevention:

Increasing one's balance may have a number of important benefits, one of the most important being the avoidance of injuries. If you have superior balance, you will have a reduced risk of injuring yourself by slipping, tripping, or falling. This is of utmost importance as you become older since slips and falls may result in serious wounds such as broken bones or brain damage. Improving your coordination and balance may dramatically lower the likelihood of being involved in one of these mishaps. You will be able to reply more quickly and effectively to changes in your surroundings if you improve your proprioception, which is your body's awareness of its location in space. This will help you avoid any mishaps that may have been avoided.

2. Postural Alignment:

Maintaining a healthy posture is essential to maintaining balance. If you have poor balance, you are more prone to adopt uncomfortable or slouched postures, which may lead to muscular imbalances and chronic discomfort if they are maintained for an extended period of time. A reduction in the likelihood of problems such as lower back pain, neck discomfort, and postural irregularities may result from improving one's balance. This helps preserve the appropriate alignment of the spine and other portions of the body.

3. Enhanced Core Strength:

It is very necessary to have a robust core in order to achieve total strength and stability. Engaging your core muscles, which comprise the muscles of your belly, lower back, and pelvis, is necessary to improve your balance. Building up the strength of these core muscles may result in improved posture, enhanced spinal health, and a lower chance of suffering from back issues. Additionally, it makes day-to-day tasks simpler and more time and effort-efficient.

4. Coordination and Agility:

A higher level of balance improves coordination and agility, both of which are essential for participating in a wide variety of bodily demanding activities. If you want to move with better comfort and elegance, whether you're engaging in sports, dancing, or even simply navigating through congested city streets, improving your balance is one of the best ways to do it. This may lead to an increase in the pleasure of activities as well as a decrease in the risk of injury when engaging in physical activity or engaging in leisure pursuits.

5. Functional Independence:

Maintaining a steady equilibrium is necessary for the completion of routine activities. Maintaining your equilibrium is necessary for activities as seemingly mundane as getting up from a chair, climbing stairs, and carrying groceries. When you work on improving your balance, you strengthen your ability to do these activities independently, which is something that becomes more crucial as you get older. It may make it easier for you to keep your independence and provide you with a better overall quality of life.

6. Athletic Performance:

Athletes in many different sports, like gymnastics and basketball, depend on balance to perform at their best. Gains in agility, accuracy, and endurance are just some of the benefits that may accrue to an athlete who works on improving their balance. Improving your balance is one of the most important things you can do to improve your performance in any sport or activity, whether you compete professionally or simply enjoy playing for fun.

7. A Speedier Recovery After Your Workout:

Your body needs rest in order to recuperate after a particularly taxing exercise or session of physical activity. Maintaining a healthy sense of balance may help speed up the healing process by lowering the probability of suffering an injury during physical activity and making certain that your muscles and joints are operating at their full potential. This, in turn, enables a speedier recovery that is also more efficient, which, in turn, enables you to go back to your exercises or hobbies sooner.

8. Methods for Reducing Stress:

A reduction in stages of stress and anxiety is another potential benefit of improved balance. The mental state may become more at ease as a result of the physical act of concentrating on balance and participating in exercises like yoga or tai chi, both of which place an emphasis on maintaining balance. These techniques serve to promote mindfulness as well as relaxation, which in turn helps to lower levels of stress and increase mental well-being.

9. Improved Capabilities of the Mind:

There is a close relationship between one's physical health and their mental sharpness. Cognitive function may be improved by participating in activities that provide a challenge to your balance, such as workouts that specifically target balance or sports like yoga and martial arts. Memory, the ability to solve problems, and the brain's general health may all be helped by engaging in these activities, which demand focus and coordination.

10. A Heightened Awareness of One's Own Body:

Enhancing one's sense of balance also contributes to a heightened awareness of one's body. You develop a greater awareness of your body, both its capabilities and its limitations. Having this level of self-awareness may assist you in making more informed decisions about mobility, physical activity, and your general health. It is also possible that it may make you more aware of the demands of your body, such as the need for proper rest and recuperation.

11. Increased Self-Assurance as a Result:

Gaining control of your balance may do wonders for your self-esteem. Having the knowledge that you have the physical potential to move with ease, do activities without the fear of falling, or thrive in physical pursuits may contribute to enhanced levels of self-assurance. This greater confidence may extend to other aspects of your life, leading to a more positive self-image and a higher overall mental well-being for you.

12. Skills for Recovering from a Fall:

Falls are always a possibility, regardless of how well one's balance may be. Having improved balance, on the other hand, may help you get back on your feet more quickly and efficiently in the event that you trip or lose your footing. You'll be able to respond to a fall and modify your body posture to lessen the force of the fall, which might help you avoid more severe injuries.

13. Advantages to Your Health Over the Long Term:

Beyond the direct advantages to one's body and mind, there are further benefits to be gained by strengthening one's balance. Maintaining a healthy equilibrium may help you stay healthy over the long run by lowering your chances of developing chronic illnesses that are linked to ageing, such as osteoporosis and cardiovascular disease. In addition to this, it helps preserve joint health, which is essential if you want to keep your mobility as you get older.

14. Interactions in Social Settings:

Attending part in activities that emphasize equilibrium may be a social experience, whether it's attending a group fitness class, joining a dancing club, or practising yoga with friends. These are all examples of activities that concentrate on equilibrium. This kind of social connection may lead to improvements in mental health and create a feeling of community as well as support for the individual.

15. A Stronger Connection Between the Mind and the Body:

Meditation and other practices that bring awareness to the mind-body connection are often included in balancing routines. This may result in a greater comprehension of how your body moves and how it feels, establishing a stronger link between your mental and physical experiences. This strengthened link between the mind and the body may be very beneficial to one's overall health.

16. Getting a Better Night's Rest:

The quality of your sleep may improve if you engage in regular physical activity, particularly activities that concentrate on your balance. It makes falling asleep easier, it keeps you sleeping for longer, and it makes you feel more refreshed when you wake up. In turn, this may lead to improvements in both one's mood and their cognitive performance.

17. Acceleration of the Metabolism:

Performing activities that focus on improving your balance might assist in speeding up your metabolism. This may lead to improved control of one's weight as well as metabolic health in general. If your body has a greater metabolic rate, it will burn calories more effectively, which will contribute to improved general health and the ability to maintain a healthy weight.

18. Improved Digestive Function:

Activities like yoga, which help improve balance, may also improve digestion when practised regularly. The digestive organs may be stimulated by certain yoga positions and stretches, which can help reduce digestive disorders such as bloating and constipation.

19. Capacity for Emotional Balance:

It is possible that improvements in your physical stability will have a beneficial effect on the emotional stability you experience. Endorphins, which are natural mood relishes, are released during regular exercise and activities that concentrate on maintaining balance. This may help minimize feelings of despair and anxiety and contribute to an emotional state that is more upbeat and pleasant.

20. Education That Lasts a Lifetime:

Maintaining your equilibrium requires a persistent effort over time. Participating in activities designed to enhance your balance will always leave you with an opportunity for personal development and expansion of knowledge. This feeling of always being able to do more for oneself may be intellectually engaging and emotionally rewarding.

Practical Tips for Improving Balance:

Now that we've discussed the many reasons why you should work on improving your balance, let's talk about some useful advice and exercises that you can do to become better at maintaining your equilibrium:

1. Exercises for Improving Your Balance:

Include workouts that specifically target your balance as part of your program. A few examples of these would include walking heel-to-toe, standing on one leg, or making use of a balance board or stability ball. Other great possibilities include tai chi, yoga, and similar practices.

2. Building Strength in the Core:

A solid core is necessary for maintaining equilibrium. Planks, Russian twists, and leg rises are all great exercises that target your core muscles and should be included in your training routine.

3. Exercises to Improve Flexibility:

Increasing your flexibility may help you maintain your balance. Include stretching exercises in your routine to improve both your range of motion and the mobility of your joints.

4. The Practices of Mindfulness:

Mindfulness and the mind-body connection are emphasized in a variety of practices, such as yoga and tai chi. These practices may help improve balance and decrease stress.

5. Keep Yourself Active:

Maintaining your equilibrium and general health via regular physical exercise, such as walking and riding, might be beneficial.

6. Keep a Balanced and Healthful Diet:

The state of one's nutrition has a substantial impact on one's entire well-being, particularly one's sense of equilibrium. It is essential to consume a diet that is both well-balanced and nourishes both the muscles and the bones.

7. Relaxation and Recuperation:

A healthy amount of sleep and time for recuperation are both necessary components of a balanced and healthy lifestyle. Be sure to get enough sleep so that your body has the opportunity to heal and replenish itself.

8. Seek the Advice of Qualified Professionals:

Consider working with a fitness expert or a physical therapist who can give tailored instruction and support if you are confused about the appropriate exercises or approaches for improving your balance.

Conclusion

Improving one's equilibrium has a wide range of benefits, some of which include enhanced physical, mental, and emotional well-being. Maintaining a sense of equilibrium throughout everyday life is essential since it has a bearing on a wide range of aspects, including the avoidance of injuries, physical performance, cognitive function, and emotional steadiness. You may enjoy these various advantages and improve your overall quality of life by adopting a healthy lifestyle, which includes the practice of mindfulness and workouts that concentrate on maintaining or restoring balance. Keep in mind that obtaining balance in your life means not just gaining bodily stability but also reaching equilibrium in all parts of your life, which will lead to a life that is both healthier and more rewarding for you.

Chapter 4: Safety Precautions

1. Provide Tips on Creating a Safe Exercise Environment at Home.

It is critical to your health, motivation, and the general effectiveness of your fitness regimen that you design an exercise space in your house that is free from potential hazards. Having a secure location in which to exercise may help you avoid injuries, enhance your self-confidence, and make your exercises at home more productive. This is true whether you are just starting out or are an experienced fitness fanatic. In this extensive guide, we will go over a variety of recommendations that can support you in creating a secure atmosphere in which to work at home.

1. Clear the Space

Getting rid of any impediments or clutter in the training space is the first thing you should do when you want to create a secure atmosphere for working out at home. This includes any and all items—furniture, carpets, or otherwise—that could get in the way of your motions while you're working out. Ensure that there is sufficient room for a variety of activities to be performed without the risk of colliding with anything. Your chances of stumbling or falling during your exercise are reduced if there isn't a lot of clutter around you.

2. Proper Lighting

During physical activity, having enough illumination is critical to ensuring one's safety. Inadequate illumination might make it difficult to view your surroundings clearly, which can make it more difficult to precisely position your body. To decrease the risk of damage and confirm that you are working out with the correct technique, you should make sure that your training space has enough lighting. Having access to natural light is preferable, but if that's not an option, consider making an investment in LED lighting that is both bright and efficient.

3. Non-Slip Flooring

It is crucial to choose a flooring material that does not slide if one wants to keep one's balance and avoid mishaps. If you are exercising on a hard floor, you may want to think about utilizing exercise mats or interlocking foam tiles. These materials not only offer cushioning but also limit the chance of sliding, which is particularly important while doing workouts that entail movement or leaping.

4. Proper Ventilation

It is essential to have enough ventilation in order to keep the area in which exercise is being performed pleasant and risk-free. During your exercises, having enough ventilation may assist in controlling the temperature and lower the likelihood that you will overheat. In addition to this, it guarantees that you will always have access to clean air, which may improve both your endurance and your ability to concentrate.

5. Access to Water

During exercise, it is essential for both your health and safety that you keep yourself well-hydrated. When you exercise at home, it is important to ensure that you have quick access to water. Maintain easy access to a bottle of water so that you may take sips whenever you feel the need, especially during more strenuous activities. During physical activity, dehydration may cause symptoms such as dizziness and weariness, both of which can be hazardous.

6. Mirror

It might be helpful to have a full-length mirror in your training room so that you can check your form and posture while you work out. Your ability to avoid injury and maximize the benefits of your workouts depends on maintaining correct form. You are able to make immediate modifications to your form and check that you are moving in the appropriate manner when you have a clear view of yourself in the mirror.

7. Emergency Plan

It is always a good idea to have an emergency plan in place, but it is more important to do so when you are exercising by yourself. Make sure that someone is aware that you are going to the gym, and follow up with them after your exercise to see how they are doing. In the event of a crisis, you should also have a phone close at hand and maintain a list of people to call in an emergency within easy reach. In a potentially life-threatening circumstance, having a plan for what to do in the event of an accident or injury may make all the difference.

8. Well-Maintained Equipment

If you workout at home, you should routinely examine and repair your exercise equipment to ensure that it is safe to use. Check that there are no loose bolts, broken pieces, or other cyphers of wear and tear. It is important to ensure that your equipment is in excellent functioning condition in order to avoid any mishaps or injuries. Adjust any loose screws, lubricate any moving parts, and replace any components that have become worn as necessary.

9. Suitable Attire

It is important to remember that wearing suitable fitness clothes is not just about looking good; it is also a safety factor. Pick up clothes and shoes that are not only comfortable but also provide the right amount of support. Depending on the sort of exercise you do, you should look for shoes that give stability, arch support, and cushioning. Avoid wearing baggy clothes since it may cause you to trip over your own equipment or hamper your mobility.

10. Stay Informed

The most effective method for guaranteeing your own personal safety when working out at home is to educate yourself. It is important to acquire the correct workout methods and form in order to limit the likelihood of injury. There is a wealth of information available to you in the shape of videos, fitness apps, and internet resources that may direct you in the proper execution of exercises. In addition, if you want individualized instruction, you might think about enrolling in online courses or working with a virtual personal trainer.

11. Warm-Up and Cool Down

Always be sure you start and end your exercises with a warm-up and a cool-down program. By properly warming up, you may better prepare your muscles and joints for activity, which in turn lowers the chance of pulling muscles and other injuries. By allowing your body to slowly return to its resting condition after exercise, cooling down may help reduce the amount of muscle discomfort experienced after a workout. The importance of correctly warming up and cooling down after exercise cannot be overstated.

12. Variety of Exercises

Not only is it excellent for your health to engage in a range of activities, but it is also beneficial for your safety. When you repeatedly work the same muscle groups, you run the risk of creating imbalances that may lead to injury. Alternate between various types of workouts in your regimen to reduce the risk of overuse injuries and boost your level of general fitness.

13. Be Mindful of Overexertion

However, in order to make improvements in your fitness level, it is essential that you do it in a manner that does not compromise your safety. Exerting oneself beyond one's capabilities might result in tiredness and may even cause damage. Pay attention to your body and learn to recognize when you need to rest. It is not in your best interest to push yourself to the point of fatigue since this might put your form and safety at risk.

14. Use Safety Measures for Cardio Workouts

When you conduct high-intensity cardio exercises at home, extra safety issues come into play, including the following:

- **Invest in a heart rate monitor**: ensure that you remain within your safe training zone. This will guarantee that you get the most out of your workouts.
- **Emergency stop:** If you are going to be utilizing a stationary bike or a treadmill, you should get acquainted with the emergency stop mechanism of the machine.
- **Sufficient distance:** Make sure there is sufficient space around your cardiovascular equipment to avoid mishaps in the event that you have to stop unexpectedly.

15. Consider a Home Gym

If you have the room and the funds, constructing a home gym may offer you an exercise setting that is both secure and handy for your workouts. You have the option of designing the area and purchasing high-quality equipment to cater to your individual requirements for physical activity. You will have more control over the atmosphere and fewer reasons to worry about your safety when you work out in your own home gym rather than a shared public facility.

16. Child and Pet Safety

If you have young children or animals in the house, making sure they are safe should also be a high concern for you. be sure that your exercise gear and accessories are out of reach, and check to be sure that they won't go in the way of your exercises. In order to decrease the risk of injury during your exercises, you should consider reserving a space that is free from potential hazards for children.

17. Stay Hygienic

Hygiene and cleanliness are more important than ever in light of recent events that have occurred on a worldwide scale. In order to stop the transmission of germs, you should clean your tools both before and after each usage. During your exercises, you should wipe down all handles, surfaces, and pieces of equipment that you come into contact with using a clean towel or disinfectant wipes.

18. Regular Maintenance

The task of keeping your workout environment in good condition is a continual one. Inspect and clean up your training room on a regular basis. When necessary, replace any flooring, matting, or equipment that has been worn out. Make sure that your lights and ventilation are operating at their optimum levels by giving them close attention. Maintaining the cleanliness of your area will ensure that you continue to work out in an atmosphere that is both secure and productive.

19. Safety Equipment

Consider including some kind of protective gear in your exercise regimen, taking into account the kinds of activities in which you engage. For instance, while lifting weights, you should use collars to keep the weights in place, and you should always have a spotter beside you when lifting high loads. When doing workouts that require you to fall or leap, you should think about utilizing crash mats or other types of safety padding.

20. Listen to Your Body

Listen to what your body is telling you to do since this is maybe the most crucial safety guideline. During your exercise, you should immediately stop if you start to feel any pain, discomfort, dizziness, or other symptoms that are out of the ordinary. Conquering the attitude of "no pain, no gain" is essential for ensuring your own safety. It is always best to err on the side of caution and seek medical counsel when necessary, especially when pushing through discomfort might result in more injuries. In conclusion, one of the most important aspects of keeping a healthy fitness program that does not result in injuries is making sure that the setting in which one exercises at home is safe. You may create an environment for working out that is conducive to your health and well-being, as well as safe and efficient, if you follow the advice in this section. Whether you're just starting out or have years of expertise under your belt, it's important to keep in mind that safety should always be your number one concern.

Chapter 5: Simple Balance Exercises

1. Introduce a Series of Basic Balance Exercises for Seniors.

It is essential for seniors to keep their balance in order to avoid falling as they become older and to continue engaging in physical activity. Exercises that focus on maintaining or improving balance are an essential component of any program designed for older adults since they assist in improving stability, lowering the chance of accidents, and boosting general mobility. In this section, we will walk you through a series of fundamental balancing exercises that have been developed particularly for older adults. Because these exercises are risk-free, efficient, and can be modified to put up a wide range of fitness levels, they are well suited for older individuals who want to improve their balance as well as their general health.

Standing on One Leg:

Standing on one leg is a basic balancing exercise that helps develop the muscles in the legs and improves overall stability. Standing on one leg also helps improve overall stability.

Instructions:

- If you feel like you need support, you may stand next to a solid chair or a wall.
- Raise one leg off the ground a few inches at a time while maintaining a straight back position.
- Your goal should be to stay balanced on one leg for twenty to thirty seconds.
- Alternate between your left and right legs and continue the workout.
- As your comfort level grows, you should gradually extend the time of the exercise.

Benefits:

- Builds up the leg muscles' strength.
- Increases one's proprioception (also known as bodily awareness).
- Increases overall sense of equilibrium.

Heel-To-Toe Walk:

You will need excellent balance and coordination to complete the heel-to-toe walk, which is also referred to as the "tightrope" walk.

Instructions:

- Maintain this position by standing with your feet together and putting one foot in front of the other.
- Take a step forward and bring the heel of one foot to the tip of the foot on the opposite side of you.

- Carry on your way, always putting one foot in front of the other as you walk in a straight path.
- If you need assistance maintaining your balance, keep your arms out to the sides.
- Take roughly ten to fifteen steps forward.

Benefits:

- Improves both your balance and your coordination.
- Improves the strength of the leg muscles.
- Enhances one's walk.

Hip Hikes:

Hip hikes are a fantastic workout for improving both the balance and the stability of the hips.

Instructions:

- If you need assistance, you may stand next to a chair or a counter.
- Raise one leg to the side while maintaining a straight stance with the other.
- Reduce the height of the elevated leg while keeping your support on the other foot.
- Continue in this manner for ten to fifteen repetitions on each side.

Benefits:

- Improves the strength of the hip muscles.
- Enhances the lateral stability of the structure.
- Improves the overall sense of equilibrium.
- Exercises Done While Standing From a Seat
- These exercises put an emphasis on rising from a sitting posture, which is a movement that is performed often in everyday life.

Instructions:

- Place both of your feet firmly on the ground and cross your arms over your chest as you take a seat on a solid chair.
- Don't use your hands to help you get up from the chair; just get up on your own.
- Begin to slowly sit back down while maintaining control of the action.
- Complete 10–15 reps of the exercise.

Benefits:

- Improves the strength of the leg muscles.
- Facilitates the movement from sitting to standing by providing additional support.
- When getting up from a chair, it provides improved balance.

- Weight Shifts:
- Weight changes are a straightforward and efficient technique for enhancing both balance and stability.

Instructions:

- Take a standing position with your feet about hip-width apart.
- Move your weight gradually from one foot to the other while elevating the heel of one foot just a little bit off the ground.
- Keep alternating your weight shifts back and forth for the next thirty seconds to one minute.
- While shifting your weight, you can try doing it with your eyes closed for an added challenge.

Benefits:

- Increases one's sense of proprioception.
- Increases the stability of the ankle.
- Improves the overall sense of equilibrium.

Tap Your Toes:

Lower body strength and stability are improved by doing toe taps, which are a low-impact form of exercise.

Instructions:

- Take a standing position with your feet about hip-width apart.
- Raise one foot off the ground and softly tap your toe in front of you, then repeat the action behind you.
- Keep going in this manner for 10-15 taps on each leg.

Benefits:

- Improves the strength of the leg muscles.
- Balance and coordination are both improved.
- Improves stability at the ankle joint.

Keeping Your Eyes Closed While Balancing on One Foot:

This exercise takes the standard "standing on one leg" exercise and raises the difficulty level by removing visual clues from the equation, making it more difficult for you to maintain your balance.

Instructions:

- If you feel like you need it, stand near to a support.
- Raise the heel of one foot just off the ground.

- Try to keep your eyes closed as you focus on keeping your balance on one leg for ten to fifteen seconds.
- Alternate between your left and right legs and continue the workout.

Benefits:

- Increases one's sense of proprioception.
- Improves the strength of the leg muscles.
- Enhances one's sense of balance in circumstances when visual input is limited.

Swinging Your Legs:

Leg swings are a great exercise for improving dynamic balance as well as flexibility.

Instructions:

- Take a position where you are facing strong support, such as a chair or a wall.
- Raise one of your legs and move it in a forward and backward motion.
- The leg swings should be repeated for 10–15 repetitions on each leg.

Benefits:

- Improves both static balance and dynamic flexibility.
- Improves strength in the thighs and hips.

The Clock Strikes:

Clock reaches are an excellent workout to stress your balance in a variety of directions since they are performed in a round motion.

Instructions:

- Balance yourself on one foot.
- Imagine that you are the pivot point in the middle of a clock.
- You may move your free foot to the various "hours" on the clock (for example, 12 o'clock, 3 o'clock, and 6 o'clock).
- Keeping each posture for a brief period of time.
- Perform this exercise on the opposite leg in the same manner.

Benefits:

- Helps improve balance as well as proprioception in a number of different ways.
- Improves the strength of the leg muscles.

Position of the Yoga Tree:

The yoga "tree pose" is an excellent balancing exercise for older citizens since it combines strength training with flexibility and balance training.

Instructions:

- Maintain this stance with your feet touching.
- Raise one foot off the ground and rest it on the inner thigh of the leg that is supporting your body, either above or below the knee.
- Put your hands together in front of your chest in the shape of a prayer.
- Put your attention on anything in front of you to help you maintain your balance.
- Maintain the situation for twenty to thirty seconds.
- The exercise is repeated using the opposite leg.

Benefits:

- Improves both your balance and your flexibility.
- Improves the strength of the leg muscles.
- Facilitates mental concentration while also calming the nerves.

Seated Arm Raises

- Take out a set of dumbbells, a resistance band, or a medicine ball.
- Sit in the chair with your hips as far back as possible. Make sure your back is firmly close to the chair's backrest.
- Maintain a tight core (abdomen and lumbar). Extend your chest.
- Keep dumbbell arms to the sides of the body, allowing them to hang naturally with both palms facing the body.
- Slide a resistance band under the chair or sit on it till it is the same distance on both sides of the body. Then, hold together arms at your sides, allowing them to hang naturally with palms towards the body.
- Place a medicine ball at the edge of your lap and grip the ball with both hands on each side.
- Continue to lift the arms up in front of the body while keeping the arms straight and palms facing forward.
- When the arms are parallel to the floor, and the hands are in direct sight of the eyes, stop the action.
- Return to the starting position gradually.

Benefits:

- Front deltoid muscle development and strengthening are aided by seated front shoulder lifts. This can improve the cosmetics of your shoulders and offer a more balanced shoulder look.
- Because it activates the stabilising muscles surrounding the shoulder joint, performing sitting front shoulder raises with appropriate form can improve shoulder stability and minimize the chance of injury.

Seated Arm Circles

- 2 minutes in length
- Sit with your back straight and your feet flat on the ground.

- Straighten your arms out to the sides.
- Begin by doing little forward arm circles.
- As you proceed, gradually increase the size of the circles.
- After 1 minute, alternate between forming backward circles and forward circles for the remaining minute.
- Seated arm circles train your upper body and shoulders, improving posture and decreasing upper body tension.

Benefits:

Seated arm circles help improve the mobility of your shoulder joints. This can be especially advantageous for persons who have tight or stiff shoulders due to sedentary lifestyles or poor posture.

Seated Back Bend

- Sit comfortably on the chair's edge. Maintain core stability by keeping the back erect and the spine square. Maintain a flat foot on the floor. Maintain this protected stance for the hips and lower body.
- Put both hands on your hips.
- Slowly arch your back inward, pulling your tummy outward, then lean backwards, utilizing only your upper body.
- Extend the back in this position till you reach a comfortable stretch.
- Hold this position for 10-20 seconds before freeing and returning to the beginning position.
- Repeat the pattern 3-5 times or as desired.

Benefits:

- Regular sitting backbends can help repair bad posture by stretching and strengthening the muscles responsible for upright posture. This can aid in the treatment of disorders such as rounded shoulders and excessive forward bending.
- Individuals suffering from mild to severe back discomfort may benefit from seated backbends. Stretching and extending the back muscles can help reduce back stress and discomfort.

Chair Push-Ups (Upper and Lower Body)

- Sit on the chair's edge, grasping the edges for support.
- Lower your chest towards the chair by sliding your hips forward and bending your elbows.
- Return to the beginning position by pushing through your hands.
- Chair push-ups should be done for 5-10 reps with controlled motions.

Benefits:

Chair pushups primarily target the muscles in your chest, shoulders, and triceps. They help build and tone these muscles, which can improve your upper body strength.

Biceps Curls

You will require A solid chair (optional) and light weights (if weights are unavailable, bottles filled with water or canned foods may suffice).

- Sit or stand by the workout chair.
- (If sitting) Feet Securely on the ground and hip-width apart.
- (If standing) Standing straight with feet hip-width apart.
- Deltoid straight.
- Arms by your sides.
- Hold the weights in both hands.
- Rise your hands in a vertical motion, up to your Deltoid, keeping the wrists straight, and inhale.
- Bring your hands downcast and exhale. (You can do this one hand at a time too).
- Replication 8-10 times.

Benefits:

- Make stronger the upper part of the arm.
- Advances gripping capacity.
- Make stronger bicep muscle tissue, which makes lifting activities easier.

Modified Chair Push-ups

- Stand up straight in front of the chair.
- Place both hands on the seat of the chair. Shift both feet backwards a few steps, keeping both arms slightly bent at the elbows till the torso is in a slanting posture in front of the chair. I checked that the buttocks are not raised up in the air and that the back is not arched. From shoulder to heel, the body should be in a straight line. If a senior feels resistance (tension) in their core, they are at the right place. The elbows should be close to the body's sides.
- Bend the elbows slowly, bringing the body closer to the chair.
- Push back to the start position after the chin has almost affected the chair (or as close to the chair as feasible).

Benefits:

Modified pushups still engage the chest, shoulders, and triceps, helping you build upper body strength. They are an excellent starting point for beginners who may still need to gain the strength to perform regular pushups.

Seated Triceps Dips

- Sit on the chair's edge with your palms on the seat next to your pelvis.

- Lower your body by sliding your pelvis off the chair and bending your forearms.
- Return to the beginning position by pushing up.
- Repeat 15-20 times.

Benefits:

- Seated tricep dips are an excellent exercise for isolating and developing the triceps brachii, a muscle near the rear of the upper arm. This can assist in enhancing your arms' overall look and strength.
- Seated tricep dips can help tone and define your triceps, making your arms seem more sculpted.

Seated Leg Extensions (Legs and Core)

- Place your feet flat on the floor and sit up straight.
- Lift one of your Limbs straight out in front of you, parallel to the ground.
- Hold for a few seconds before lowering it again.
- Rep with the opposite leg.

Benefits:

Seated leg lifts target the major muscles of your legs, helping to build strength in your quadriceps, hamstrings, and hip flexors. This can be particularly advantageous for persons looking to improve their lower body strength.

Sit to Stands

- Place your feet on the edge of the seat and sit comfortably.
- Maintain a tight core (abdomen and lumbar). Spread your chest.
- Maintain a relaxed situation in the forward-facing of the body with both hands in front of the body in a comfortable stance for balance.
- Sit up slowly from the chair until you are completely standing. When transitioning from sitting to standing up, be sure your knees aren't bowing inward; instead, they should be extending outward from the centre of your body. This exercise entails thrusting the body to a standup posture with the hips rather than the knees.
- Return to the start posture while checking for proper knee placement.

Benefits:

Sit-to-stand exercises primarily target the muscles in your legs, including the quadriceps, hamstrings, and calf muscles. Regularly performing these exercises can help improve leg strength, which is vital for activities like walking, climbing stairs, and maintaining balance.

Heel Slides

- Place your feet on the edge of the seat and sit comfortably.

- Maintain a tight core (abdomen and lumbar). Spread your chest.
- To maintain stability, place equal hands on the sides of the sitting chair and grab the seat.
- Extend one leg in front of you and point your toes frontward. The foot of the stretched leg should be diagonal to the hips. Place the foot on the upper of a blanket or other material if using one.
- The 2nd leg should be bent naturally, close to the torso, and placed on the floor.
- Keep a flat foot with the prolonged leg, push in contrast to the home floor, and draw the foot gently toward the body until it reaches the flexed position of the opposite leg.
- Extend the leg back to the beginning position while maintaining pressure.
- A single rep is when you complete the whole process of pulling and pushing your foot back to the beginning position.

Benefits:

- Heel slides are effective in improving joint mobility, particularly in the hip and knee joints. They help increase the range of motion, making it relaxed for individuals to perform daily activities and functional movements.
- Regularly performing heel slides can help increase the flexibility of the body muscles, tendons, and ligaments around the hip and knee joints. This improved flexibility can reduce the risk of injury and improve overall joint health.

Conclusion

For elders to live an active lifestyle without risking injury, it is necessary for them to have a proper balance. The sequence of fundamental balancing exercises that we have shown in this book is intended to assist elderly citizens in enhancing their stability, reducing the risk of falling, and maintaining their confidence in their day-to-day activities. Keep in mind that consistency is the most important factor; doing these workouts on a regular basis will provide the finest outcomes. In addition, you should always put your safety first, seek assistance when it is required of you, and talk to a medical expert if you have any special concerns about your health. Starting off at your own speed and progressively increasing the difficulty of the exercises as you gain confidence in your skill to maintain your balance is essential to the success of any fitness program. These activities will not only progress your physical well-being but will also contribute to a life in your elderly years that is more independent and enjoyable.

Chapter 6: Balance Routines

1. Cater to Different Fitness Levels and Specific Goals.

How Online Fitness Coaches Cater to Different Fitness Levels and Goals

Online fitness coaching has grown in popularity among fitness lovers of all levels in recent years. With the ease and low cost of virtual training, an increasing number of people are seeking the advice and assistance of online fitness instructors to help them accomplish their fitness objectives. However, what does it mean to cater to various fitness levels and goals in an online setting? Let us investigate more.

Understanding Different Fitness Levels and Goals

Fitness is a journey that begins with one step. Whether you're a beginner or a seasoned athlete, online coach fitness can give instruction and support to help you reach your objectives. In this post, we'll look at the various fitness levels and typical goals that online trainers may help with.

Beginner Fitness Levels

It might be difficult to know where to begin if you are new to exercise. This is where online coaches can help. They may offer essential advice on good form and technique to avoid injury and lay a firm basis for future growth. Bodyweight exercises are frequently used in beginner-focused workouts to assist in improving strength and mobility before adding more complicated motions and weights. Online coaches may also aid you with nutrition to fuel your body for peak performance.

Intermediate Fitness Levels

Intermediate-level customers often have some exercise experience and may want to improve their strength and endurance while growing muscle. Online coaches may offer individualized programming to assist customers in reaching their unique objectives while also challenging them with new exercises and training strategies on a regular basis. They can also advise customers on injury prevention and recovery to help them stay healthy and avoid setbacks.

Advanced Fitness Levels

Advanced customers already have a solid fitness foundation and may be competing in events or striving for high levels of performance. Online coaches can assist these customers in realizing their maximum potential by using high-level programming and training strategies. They can also advise customers on sports psychology and mental preparation to help them perform well under duress.

Common Fitness Goals

Online trainers cater to a number of typical fitness goals in addition to different fitness levels. Weight loss, muscle growth, injury recovery, and sport-specific performance enhancement are all possibilities. Coaches can modify their programming to assist clients in reaching their unique goals while remaining motivated. They can also help customers remain on track and achieve progress by providing responsibility and support. Overall, online coaching may be a very beneficial tool for anybody trying to improve their fitness. You can reach your objectives and become the greatest version of yourself with specialized coaching and support.

The Role of Online Fitness Coaches

Online fitness coaching has changed the way people think about their health and fitness objectives. With the advancement of technology, it is now simpler than ever to work with a coach remotely, providing greater flexibility and accessibility. The following are some of the primary advantages of working with an online fitness coach:

Personalized Workout Plans

One of the primary advantages of online fitness coaching is the opportunity to create customized training regimens for each client. Coaches can use individual goals, fitness levels, and equipment availability to design a program that maximizes performance while minimizing injury risk. This implies that customers may have a fitness regimen that is customized to their unique requirements and tastes. For example, if a client has a history of knee issues, an online coach can design a program that avoids activities that could irritate the knee and instead focus on strengthening the muscles surrounding it. Alternatively, if a client wants to run a marathon, the coach can design a program that progressively builds distance and combines certain forms of training to enhance endurance. Click here to learn more about How to Choose the Best Online Personal Trainer in Australia.

Nutritional Guidance and Support

In addition to training regimens, online coaches can offer dietary advice and assistance to customers in order to help them accomplish their goals. Meal planning, accountability check-ins, and instruction on adequate nutrient consumption may be included to support optimal performance and wellness. A coach, for example, may provide a client with a meal plan based on their individual nutritional needs and interests. They may also advise on serving sizes, macronutrient ratios, and hydration. Coaches may help clients achieve long-term dietary adjustments that support their overall health and fitness objectives by giving this sort of assistance.

Accountability and Motivation

Online coaches may be a great source of accountability and inspiration. Even when things become rough, daily check-ins, progress monitoring, and encouragement may help clients stay on track and dedicated to their goals. A coach, for example, may send a client a daily message asking how their training went or encouraging them. They may also use images, measurements, or performance indicators to track progress. Coaches may help clients stay motivated and accountable to their goals by giving this sort of assistance.

Progress Tracking and Adjustments

Online coaches may track their customers' progress toward their goals and make required changes to their programming to ensure continuous success. Changing workouts or increasing difficulty levels may be used to assist clients in breaking through plateaus and attaining new levels of fitness. For example, if a client has been performing the same routine for several weeks and isn't seeing results, the coach may change the program to incorporate more difficult exercises or raise the weight or reps. Coaches may help customers show progress and achieve their goals by making these modifications.

Catering to Individual Needs and Preferences

There is no such thing as a one-size-fits-all strategy to exercise. Everyone has different requirements and interests, and online coaches are aware of this. As a result, they provide bespoke training that can be custom-made to each customer's specific requirements.

Adapting Workouts for Different Abilities

Online coaches may also modify exercises to accommodate differing abilities, ensuring that all customers can participate and profit from the programming. Customers with injuries or limits may require modifications, while advanced customers may require progressions. This implies that an online coach can assist you no matter where you are on your fitness journey. If you have a knee injury that precludes you from practising high-impact exercises, for example, your coach can tweak your routines to incorporate low-impact options that still challenge you and help you grow. If you're an experienced athlete wishing to increase your training, your coach can give advanced routines and programming that will push you to your limits.

Incorporating Personal Interests and Hobbies

The option to combine personal interests and hobbies into your training is one of the most significant advantages of online coaching. Fitness does not have to be a chore, and coaches may help clients find activities that they actually like. If you enjoy hiking or rock climbing, for example, your coach can include these activities in your training plan to help you improve strength and endurance for those sports. Alternatively, if you prefer dance or yoga, your coach can design exercises that include those motions and styles.

Addressing Specific Health Concerns

Online coaches can give personalized programming and support to customers with specific health issues, such as diabetes or heart disease, to help manage these diseases while still accomplishing fitness objectives. This is especially relevant because exercise has been shown to be an effective technique for controlling and preventing chronic illnesses. If you have diabetes, for example, your coach can design a training regimen that helps manage your blood sugar levels and raises insulin sensitivity. If you have heart disease, your coach can include cardiovascular activities that can improve your heart health and lower your risk of future cardiac events.

Balancing Time Constraints and Commitments

Finally, online coaches may help customers manage their time obligations and limits. Coaches may give efficient and effective training programming that fits into each client's specific lifestyle and schedule, whether it's a demanding job schedule or family responsibilities. For example, if you only have 30 minutes to exercise every day, your coach may design a high-intensity interval training (HIIT) session that makes the most of your time while still producing results. If you travel regularly for work, your coach can design bodyweight exercises that you can perform without any equipment in your hotel room. Overall, online coaching provides a degree of customization and flexibility that typical gym environments can not provide. You may reach your fitness objectives in a pleasant, sustainable, and successful manner by working with a coach who understands your unique requirements and preferences.

The Bottom Line

Online fitness coaching has grown in popularity in recent years and with good cause. It provides people with a simple and effective option to attain their fitness objectives, regardless of their location, schedule, or fitness level. One of the most significant advantages of online fitness coaching is the customized programming that customers receive. Online trainers, as opposed to generic fitness programs seen in publications or online, design personalized regimens geared to each client's particular requirements and goals. As a result, customers may achieve progress more quickly and effectively than they would with a one-size-fits-all strategy. In addition to tailored training, online coaches offer nutritional advice to assist customers in properly feeding their bodies. This is especially crucial for persons who are new to exercise or have previously struggled with weight control. Clients may improve their workout outcomes by learning how to make good food choices and properly feed their bodies. However, one of the most significant features of online fitness coaching is the motivational assistance provided to customers. Throughout their fitness journey, online coaches will encourage, motivate, and hold customers responsible. This may make all the difference in assisting customers to remain consistent and devoted to their goals, even when life becomes hectic or difficult. Overall, online fitness coaching is an excellent resource for anybody seeking to improve their fitness and live a better lifestyle. Online coaches may assist customers in reaching new levels of fitness and achieving their objectives by providing tailored programming, dietary guidance, and motivational support.

Chapter 7: Incorporating Balance into Daily Life

1. Provide Tips on Maintaining and Enhancing Balance Throughout the Day.

Introduction

Balance is an important component of our everyday lives, influencing everything from mobility to general well-being. Maintaining and improving balance is especially important for seniors who want to dodge falls and stay active. Balance, on the other hand, isn't something we should just focus on during workouts; it's a talent that can be honed and integrated into our daily lives. In this book, we will look at tactics and ideas for maintaining and improving balance throughout the day, creating a healthier and more balanced lifestyle.

Stay Active

One of the most effective methods to enhance balance is via physical exercise. Walking, swimming, and yoga, for example, can assist in strengthening the muscles that maintain balance. Aim for at least 150 minutes per week of modest-intensity aerobic exercise, as well as muscle-strengthening activities, on two or more days each week.

Functional Movements

Concentrate on exercises and motions that mirror daily tasks. Standing on one leg, stepping over barriers, or rising from a sitting position are all examples of this. You may improve your balance in real-life circumstances by implementing these practical motions into your everyday routine.

Proper Footwear

Wearing the right footwear is critical for maintaining balance. Choose shoes with non-slip soles and adequate arch support. High heels and flip-flops should be avoided since they might increase the danger of a fall. Check the fit of your shoes and replace them when they exhibit indications of wear and tear.

Mindful Walking

Pay attention to how you walk. Lift your feet rather than shuffling, and take deliberate steps. To preserve good posture, look ahead rather than down. This attentive walking method might help you improve your balance and avoid stumbling.

Core Strength

A strong core is vital for maintaining balance. Incorporate core-strengthening exercises such as planks, bridges, and leg lifts into your program. A strong core stabilizes your body and promotes balance.

Hip Flexibility

Stretches and exercises can help you improve your hip flexibility. Hip flexibility makes it simpler to maintain balance in a variety of settings. Yoga and stretches, such as hip flexor stretches, can be extremely beneficial.

Stairs with Caution

Always use the railing for assistance when using the stairs. Take your time and use caution. Ascend or descend one step at a time, totally lifting your feet off each step before proceeding to the next.

Mind-Body Practices

Mindfulness-based therapies such as yoga and tai chi can help improve balance dramatically. These exercises emphasize body awareness, posture, and regulated movements, which can help you become more aware of your body's location in space.

Maintain Proper Posture

Balance requires proper posture. Maintain proper posture by keeping your head over your shoulder joint and your shoulders over your hips. Avoid slouching or leaning forward since this might throw your balance off.

Stay Hydrated

Dizziness and unsteadiness can result from dehydration. Drink enough water throughout the day to keep your body functioning properly, including your balance.

Balanced Diet

A healthy diet rich in key minerals, together with calcium and vitamin D, is energetic for bone health. Strong bones provide a solid basis for balance.

Regular Health Check-ups

Regular check-ups with your healthcare practitioner are critical for addressing any underlying health disorders that may influence balance, such as inner ear troubles, vision problems, or drug side effects.

Use Assistive Devices When Needed

If you're in danger of falling, don't be afraid to utilize supportive equipment like canes or walkers. These tools can help to increase stability and safety.

Home Safety

Make sure your house is clear of tripping risks. Remove any loose carpets, debris, or extension wires from walkways. Install non-slip mats in the bathroom and railings in locations where you may want assistance.

Fall Prevention Awareness

Be mindful of your surroundings and any threats. Keep an eye out for damp or slippery floors, uneven surfaces, and ice sidewalks, for example. You may avoid accidents by taking measures and making modifications.

Vision Care

Regular eye exams are essential for maintaining excellent eyesight. Poor eyesight can impair your impression of space and cause balance problems.

Balance Challenges

Incorporate balancing exercises into your everyday routine. For example, try brushing your teeth on one leg or shutting your eyes for a few seconds. These little issues might have a significant impact over time.

Adaptive Strategies

Consider adaptive solutions if you have a specific ailment that impacts your balance. If you suffer peripheral neuropathy, for example, a walking stick may give additional assistance.

Social Activities

Participate in balance-related social activities and hobbies such as dance, group exercise programs, or even gardening. Social activities not only stimulate the mind but also aid in the maintenance of bodily equilibrium.

Balance Training Devices

Use balance training items such as balance boards or stability balls. These tools can support you in advancing your balance in a safe atmosphere.

Mindfulness Meditation

Mindfulness meditation can support you in becoming more aware of your body's feelings and emotions. It may also lower tension and anxiety, which can have an indirect impact on balance.

Conclusion

Maintaining and improving balance is a continual effort that, regardless of age, may considerably improve your quality of life. By adopting the concepts and tactics discussed in this guide into your daily routine, you may provide a more solid foundation for all of your activities. Remember that balance encompasses not just physical strength but also mental awareness and lifestyle choices. With commitment and consistency, you may experience better balance, a lower chance of falling, and a more confident and meaningful life.

Chapter 8: Nutrition and Balance

1. Explore the Link Between Nutrition and Balance.

The connection between proper diet and maintaining a healthy equilibrium is a multi-faceted and essential component of human health and well-being. In the context of this discussion, the concept of balance refers to both the mental and emotional steadiness of an individual in addition to the physiological and biochemical equilibrium that exists inside the body. The provision of enough nourishment is of critical importance in maintaining this balance. In this piece, we will investigate the complex link that exists between nutrition and equilibrium, focusing on both the physical and mental elements of this connection.

Physical Balance and Nutrition:

1. Macronutrients and Energy Balance

Keeping an adequate energy balance is the cornerstone of achieving and sustaining bodily equilibrium. In order for our bodies to carry out their everyday duties and keep their numerous physiological systems running smoothly, they need a specific quantity of energy. These macronutrients, which include carbs, proteins, and fats, are the source of this energy. A diet that has the appropriate amount of each of these macronutrients in the appropriate proportions is vital for maintaining adequate amounts of energy and for good health in general.

- Carbohydrates are not only a rapid source of energy but also essential to the proper functioning of the brain. Consuming the appropriate kinds of carbs, such as whole grains and fruits, may assist in controlling one's blood sugar levels and give continuous energy throughout the day.
- Proteins are the fundamental components of our bodies and play an essential part in the process of repairing and maintaining our muscles. A diet that is well-rounded and contains an adequate amount of protein maintains normal muscular function, which is vital for maintaining balance and stability.
- Fats, particularly healthy unsaturated fats, are required for a variety of body processes, such as the absorption of fat-soluble vitamins and the maintenance of the structure of cells. These fats provide a reliable source of energy that may be used over a prolonged period of time.

2. Micronutrients and Balance

In addition to macronutrients, maintaining a healthy physical balance also requires enough consumption of micronutrients, which include things like vitamins and minerals. When critical micronutrients are not consumed in sufficient quantities, it may lead to a variety of health problems that upset the homeostasis of the body.

- Vitamin D is dangerous to maintaining strong bones as well as proper muscular function. A deficit may result in muscular weakness, which raises the risk of injuries and accidents caused by falling.
- Calcium, in conjunction with vitamin D, is an essential element in the upkeep of healthy bones. In order to avoid illnesses such as osteoporosis, which may alter one's balance and lead to fractures, it is vital to consume an adequate amount of calcium in a balanced diet.
- Magnesium is yet another mineral that contributes to the proper functioning of muscles and might influence one's equilibrium. Muscle cramps and spasms are symptoms of a deficit, which may contribute to an unstable physical state.
- Potassium plays an energetic role in the functioning of nerves and muscles. The inability to maintain one's bodily equilibrium as a result of muscular weakness and cramping might be caused by an imbalance in potassium levels.
- Vitamin B12 is energetic for maintaining healthy nerves and may also have an effect on balance. A lack of this vitamin may result in peripheral neuropathy, which can cause tingling and a loss of feeling in the feet and legs, eventually compromising a person's ability to maintain their balance.

3. Hydration and Electrolyte Balance

Maintaining a healthy level of hydration is a crucial component of overall bodily equilibrium. Water is required for a variety of processes inside the body, and a healthy electrolyte balance is important for proper muscle function and nerve communication. Water is also required for several purposes.

- Sodium, potassium, and chloride are examples of electrolytes that play a role in the body's ability to keep its fluid levels in check. Muscle weakness, cramping, and poor nerve function are all symptoms that may come from an electrolyte imbalance, and all of these symptoms can have an effect on balance.
- Because dehydration may cause symptoms such as lightheadedness, weakness, and even fainting, it is an important consideration in preserving one's equilibrium. It is also possible for it to impair cognitive function, which further increases the risk of accidents and falls.

4. Weight Management and Balance

Controlling one's weight is another essential component of having a healthy physical balance. An unhealthy amount of body fat may put pressure on both the joints and the muscles, which can result in an increased risk of falling and being injured. In addition to engaging in consistent physical exercise, getting the right diet is one of the most important factors in obtaining and keeping a healthy weight.

Mental and Emotional Balance and Nutrition

The influence that one's diet has on one's mental and emotional well-being is becoming an increasingly hot topic of study. Although it only accounts for a very small part of our total body weight, the brain consumes a significant chunk of the total amount of energy that we take in each day. The nutrients that we take in have an immediate effect on the functioning of our brains and, as a consequence, on our mental and emotional health.

1. Brain Health and Nutrients

- Omega-3 fatty acids, which may be found in fatty fish as well as in select plant sources such as flaxseeds and walnuts, are essential for maintaining healthy brain function. They are known to be beneficial to cognitive function and may assist in the prevention of mood disorders such as anxiety and depression.
- Antioxidants, for example, vitamins c and e, may assist in protecting brain cells from the damaging effects of oxidative pressure, which has been associated with declining cognitive function as well as a variety of problems relating to mental health.
- The making of neurotransmitters like serotonin and dopamine, which play an important role in the regulation of mood, requires the B vitamins, notably folate (vitamin B9) and vitamin B12. These vitamins are required for the development of these neurotransmitters.

2. Blood Sugar and Mood

It is widely established that one's mood may be significantly affected by one's blood sugar levels. Consuming foods with a high glycemic index might promote mood swings and irritation because these meals generate fast increases and dips in blood sugar. The maintenance of an unchanging blood sugar level via the consumption of a nutritionally sound diet may assist in the regulation of mood and emotions.

3. Gut-Brain Connection

Recent studies have shed light on the relationship between the stomach and the brain, leading researchers to hypothesize that the state of our gut microbiota might have an effect on our mental and emotional well-being. A healthy gut, which may be supported by a diet high in fibre, prebiotics, and probiotics, may have a good influence on mood and may minimize the risk of illnesses such as depression and anxiety.

4. Inflammation and Mental Health

Researchers have found a connection between chronic inflammation and a variety of psychological health issues, including anxiety and sadness. Anti-inflammatory foods, including fruits, vegetables, and certain spices, might possibly assist in moderating the effects of inflammation on mental well-being. Nutrition plays a crucial part in the regulation of inflammation, and this function is modulated by nutrition.

The Role of Balance in Nutrition

The concept of nutritional balance refers not only to the distribution of specific nutrients within one's diet but also to the diet as a whole. A portion of healthy food should contain a wide variety of meals coming from a number of food categories since this will provide the body with a wide range of nutrients. Additionally, it should take into consideration the individual's age, level of exercise, and demands.

1. The Role of Moderation

Consuming food in an appropriate amount is essential to achieving a nutritionally sound balance. An excessive amount of any nutrient may cause an imbalance, whether it's an excessive amount of sugar that causes spikes in blood sugar or an excessive amount of salt that affects electrolyte balance. It is very necessary for one's general health to find the optimal proportions of the various nutrients.

2. Nutrient Timing

The time when nutrients are consumed is also a very important factor. Eating at set intervals and coordinating mealtimes with your exercise schedule will help you keep your energy levels stable and support your overall physical balance. In addition, the time of nutrient consumption may have an effect on mental alertness as well as the management of mood.

3. Personalized Nutrition

Because everyone has different dietary requirements, there is no universally applicable method for achieving a healthy, well-rounded diet. When formulating a plan for a balanced diet, it is important to take into account a variety of factors, including an individual's age, gender, level of activity, and preexisting medical issues. Consultation with a qualified dietitian or nutritionist may assist in adapting dietary suggestions to the requirements of a particular individual.

4. Balance in Dietary Patterns

A variety of diet plans, such as Mediterranean food, DASH (Dietary Approaches to Stop Hypertension), and plant-based diets, place an emphasis on consuming an appropriate proportion of nutrients derived from each of the food categories. These patterns have been linked to enhanced health outcomes and may serve as useful guides towards establishing a nutritional equilibrium.

In conclusion, there is no denying the connection that exists between nutrition and equilibrium. Consuming a broad range of meals that are rich in important nutrients allows for proper nutrition, which is necessary for the maintenance of bodily stability, mental and emotional well-being, and general health. To achieve nutritional equilibrium, one must take a comprehensive strategy that takes into account not just macronutrients and micronutrients but also hydration, weight control, and customized eating habits. We may improve our quality of life and encourage balance in our lives by paying attention to the foods we consume and how those foods influence both our bodies and our thoughts.

<u>Conclusion</u>

As you near the end of the book "Senior Strength: Enhance Stability, Prevent Falls, and Boost Posture with Easy At-Home Workouts," you will see that the author has emphasized the importance of maintaining good posture. I really hope you've realized that age is nothing more than a number and not a roadblock in your life. This e-book was written with the intention of serving as a guide and a travel companion for you on the journey toward a more robust, self-assured, and healthy version of yourself in your senior years. It is not about seeming to be a bodybuilder or a fitness model; rather, it is about experiencing feelings of strength, security, and independence. In the chapters that came before this one, we dove deep into the foundations of senior strength training and investigated the many advantages that it provides. We have covered the science underlying ageing, the impacts of muscle loss and bone density reduction, as well as the impact of regular, easy-to-follow exercises that can be done at home, and how these effects may be mitigated. Because we want to make sure that your trip to improved health and vitality is as easy as it can possibly be, we have given you comprehensive exercise regimens that include not only precise directions but also examples of each step. However, the success of this eBook is entirely dependent on your dedication to bettering yourself. Keep in mind that you have the potential to make positive changes in your life, including enhancing your posture, preventing falls, and improving your balance and stability. You are making an investment in a better future with each and every tiny step you take, including every time you choose to work out or make a decision about your food that is healthy. It is essential to take time along the journey to acknowledge and appreciate your achievements. Recognize the little accomplishments that have been accomplished since they will eventually add up to big progress. Milestones include the first time you successfully finish an exercise that you previously found difficult, the instant you notice greater energy levels and better posture, and the day you confidently walk a flight of stairs without hesitation. Each of these achievements is worthy of your pride. These are the building blocks that will get you to a healthier and more vibrant version of yourself. However, we must not overlook the need to maintain consistency. It is vital to achieve one's goals. Maintaining the gains you've achieved so far will be easier if you make senior strength training a consistent part of your lifestyle. Recognize that there may likely be times when your motivation wanes and that this is a totally natural occurrence. On days like these, you should go back to this eBook, reignite your desire, and find inspiration in the experiences of those who have achieved success. Keep in mind that you are not travelling this path by yourself. Talk about it with your loved ones, your close friends, or someone you work out with. A major source of motivation may come from the support and encouragement of loved ones. In addition, if you want your exercise regimen to be tailored to your specific requirements and capabilities, you might think about getting the advice of a fitness or medical specialist. Know that your dedication to senior strength is an investment in your future, one that will give a precious return for you in the shape of better health, enhanced stability, and more confidence as we get to the end of our trip. Embrace the golden years of your life with poise and power, and may this eBook serve as your reliable companion on the journey there. We are grateful that you have decided to travel this path toward a healthier, happier, and more vibrant version of yourself with "Senior Strength" as your travelling partner. Your future seems promising, and your strength has no limits to speak of. Now, go out there and make the most of each precious minute that makes up this beautiful trip we call life.

www.ingramcontent.com/pod-product-compliance
Lightning Source LLC
Chambersburg PA
CBHW080732260726
48660CB00010B/3811